MS MADE SIMPLE

MS MADE SIMPLE

The Essential Guide to Understanding
Your Multiple Sclerosis Diagnosis

MITZI JOI WILLIAMS, MD

purposely created
PUBLISHING

MS MADE SIMPLE

Published by Purposely Created Publishing Group™

Copyright © 2019 Mitzi Joi Williams

Printed in the United States of America

ISBN: 978-1-64484-022-1

Special discounts are available on bulk quantity purchases by book clubs, associations and special interest groups. For details email: sales@publishyourgift.com or call (888) 949-6228.

For information logon to:
www.PublishYourGift.com

This book is dedicated to the many wonderful people who allow me to be a part of their "family" and take part in this journey called MS with them. We laugh, we cry, we hope, we pray, and we dream together. It will always be my privilege and honor to serve you.

TABLE OF CONTENTS

ACKNOWLEDGMENTS

I want to thank my wonderful husband Bernard for being my prayer partner, my sounding board, and my biggest cheerleader during this process. I'm also grateful for my children Sara and Chase, who gave Mommy the time and space to be creative. I am eternally grateful for my "village," including my mother, my granny, my brother, and my mother-in-law and father-in-law, for their support and encouragement, as well as for babysitting! Thank you for sharing ideas, offering feedback, and giving me the time and space to finish this project!

My thanks go to my special friends, Pam, Lauren, and Erica, for reading this work and giving me honest feedback. I also want to thank my mentor and friend Dr. Mary Hughes for introducing me to the field of MS and providing a great example of how to be authentic and provide compassionate care for those I serve.

Finally, I want to thank my amazing coaches, Dr. Draion Burch and Dr. Toni Haley, for believing in me, pushing me, and continuing to see the greatness in me.

INTRODUCTION

Like many other experiences in my life, my journey to becoming a neurologist and multiple sclerosis (MS) specialist started with a leap of faith. For the majority of my high school career, I actually wanted to be a lawyer. I read suspense novels while envisioning myself in the courtroom winning all the tough cases, but I had no idea what a legal career actually entailed. I did, however, have an amazing dentist (who I saw frequently due to my love of candy, which led to many cavities), Dr. Glen, who encouraged me to consider a career in healthcare. With his influence, as well as the support of my family, I finally decided to become a physician.

While obtaining my undergraduate degree in neuroscience and behavioral biology, I took a class called "Drugs and Behavior." While some students were a bit more focused on learning about the drugs, I listened intently as my professor discussed how the interactions between our brains and various chemicals affect different aspects of our behavior.

During my first two years of medical school, I enjoyed learning about the anatomy and function of the nervous system. I found it fascinating that neurology was a bit like the detective work in my favorite mystery novels. You start with the "problem" (symptoms) and trace the steps backward to the culprit or site of the original damage. I soon decided that I wanted to learn more about neurology.

During the third year of medical school, students do clinical rotations, which expose them to different areas of medicine and help them decide which field they may want as a career. Unfortunately, my medical school did not offer a neurology rotation during the third year, which meant I didn't actually see any neurology patients before I applied for residency. I filled out all my applications and wrote my essay about why I wanted to be a neurologist without ever having seen a neurology patient. Fortunately for me, once I started working in the field, I loved it even more than I imagined I would!

During residency, I had the amazing good fortune of working in an MS clinic with Dr. Mary Hughes, who is now both a mentor and friend. During that time, I enjoyed becoming a part of people's lives and families during their journeys with MS. I also enjoyed the challenge of treating MS, because everyone is unique and there is no "one size fits all" treatment paradigm. This newly discovered passion led me to pursue further training to become an MS specialist and embark on my next adventure.

I have had hundreds of people sit across from me in all stages of life with multiple sclerosis, ranging from those with a brand-new diagnosis to those who have been living with the condition for decades. I always ask my new patients the question: "What is MS?" It is surprising and disheartening that many who have lived with their diagnosis for years still do not understand it, or are unable to convey a basic idea of what their condition means. My passion to educate and increase knowledge in the community started in the exam room and has been going strong since that time. My desire to help and encourage those living with this condition was further fueled by the diagnosis of a family member with MS. As a physician, I continue to encourage those affected by MS to understand the condition to the best of their ability and to develop treatment goals with their healthcare team.

I have learned so much over the past ten years in practice, but I have a long way to go. I believe it is imperative that we physicians work *with* you, our patients, to develop plans to attack and treat this disease. I am an expert in MS, but you are the expert about your own body and how you feel on a daily basis. I hope that this information will answer some questions about MS and will act as a tool to prompt discussion from patients and families who need clear information about this disease. Some of this information may be new to you, or all of it may be review, but my hope is that you glean something that can help in your journey with MS.

CHAPTER 1

....

WHAT DO YOU MEAN I HAVE MULTIPLE SCLEROSIS?

If you have ever been told "You have multiple sclerosis," then you know that these four words have the power to change your life completely. The diagnosis can be devastating when unexpected, but can also be a relief to someone who has been seeking answers for symptoms and issues that suddenly interrupted life as they knew it. The diagnosis engenders fear in some and hopelessness in others. But what is MS? What does that mean?

Multiple sclerosis is the second leading cause of non-traumatic neurologic disability in young people, after motor vehicle accidents. While many individuals and charitable organizations have done a great job of raising awareness about MS in recent years, which may cause some to think it is a modern condition, MS has actually been described in medical literature since the late 1800s.

Dr. Jean-Martin Charcot, who is widely considered the "father of neurology," was one of the first scientists to piece together the description of the symptoms with the "lesions" or white spots in the brain. Furthermore, there are reports that recurrent neurological symptoms typical of multiple sclerosis were recorded in personal journals as early as the 1400s. Many discoveries and breakthroughs have been made over the years, but there is much that we still need to learn.

MS is currently considered an autoimmune disease. This means that the immune system, which normally attacks viruses and bacteria and does surveillance to keep our cells growing properly, gets confused and attacks a good, healthy part of the body. Other commonly recognized autoimmune diseases include lupus, rheumatoid arthritis, and some forms of thyroid disease. Each autoimmune disease has a different "target" or area of the body that it affects, with some affecting several parts of the body.

The "target of attack" in MS is myelin, a fatty substance that covers many of the nerves. The nerves in the central nervous system, which includes the brain, the spinal cord, and the nerves to the eyes (optic nerves), are affected specifically. Myelin helps speed up the conduction of the nerve signals, and when nerves work properly, you can move and do the things you want when you decide to do them. When the signals are interrupted by damage to the myelin, the signals "slow down," and if the damage is severe, the signals may not work at all. The removal of myelin is called "demyelination." When your doctor looks at your MRIs and refers to "white matter lesions" or "white spots," these areas represent the absence of myelin, which shows up "white" on those imaging studies. Some areas of the central nervous system are more sensitive, and thus demyelination in these areas is more likely to cause symptoms, while other areas are less so. For instance, damage to the optic nerves can result in visual loss, and spinal cord lesions can result in numbness and tingling or weakness. The signs and symptoms you get with MS depend on where the damage has been done.

"But, Dr. Williams, how did I get MS? Nobody in my family has it or has even heard of it!" I have heard this more times than I can count. The honest answer is that we don't know the cause of MS. However, we have identified several risk factors. It is likely that some combination of these risk factors, along with genetic and environmental factors, can lead to one person developing MS while another may not. There are some risk factors that are "modifiable" and some that are not.

Modifiable risk factors are ones that you can do something about. These include low vitamin D levels and cigarette smoking. Vitamin D has been a hot topic in the field of MS for several years, and there is a growing body of research exploring how vitamin D deficiency relates to the onset of MS and possibly influences the long-term course of MS. There is also concern that low vitamin D levels may increase the risk for clinical relapses. Although studies suggest that people with low vitamin D are at increased risk for MS, not everyone who has vitamin D deficiency (which is just about EVERYBODY) develops MS.

Smoking is a risk factor for many diseases, including different forms of lung disease and cancer. Smokers may have a 1.5 times higher risk of developing MS than non-smokers. There is also research suggesting that smokers may have a higher risk of relapse and a worse disease course, including faster development of secondary progressive MS. After diagnosis, people often ask what they can do to improve their health or decrease the risk of worsening their MS. The best answer to that is to quit smoking.

Genetics play a part in the development of MS, but genes don't tell the whole story. Unlike sickle cell disease, MS is not directly inherited. With sickle cell disease, if the mom has a certain gene abnormality and the dad has the same abnormality, we can predict that 1 in 4 of their kids may have the disease. The genetic factors that increase risk for MS are very complex and not as predictable. There are over two hundred different genes with various functions that are related to increased risk, and the specific roles of those genes remain unclear. The risk for MS in the general population is roughly 1 in 750 people. If you have a first-degree relative (a parent or sibling) with MS, your risk is increased, but is still low overall.

Let's look at another example. Twins are commonly studied when attempting to determine the genetic components of health because identical twins have the same DNA. Twin studies in MS showed that if one sibling developed the disease, there was only about a 25 percent chance that the other twin would also develop MS. The bottom line is, while there are some families with several close relatives with multiple sclerosis or where autoimmune disease seems to run in the family, there are also many families where a single individual may be the only person in the family with multiple sclerosis. A few years ago at a national meeting, I attended an interesting and complicated talk about the many genetic discoveries related to MS. I sat for an hour and listened to all the amazing breakthroughs about genetics and risk, but the conclusion was that we don't know what many of the genes do or how they affect the risk for developing MS. The bottom line is that we still have A LOT to learn.

Another possible environmental risk factor involves contracting viruses. There seems to be a higher risk of MS in those exposed to Epstein-Barr virus, which causes mononucleosis—what we used to call the "kissing disease" when I was in high school. Kids missed a few weeks of school due to severe fatigue and illness. Also, there is a category of medications used to treat some rheumatologic conditions that can "unmask" symptoms of MS, but these medications are not thought to cause the disease. Many people ask if there is anything that they "did" to bring on the disease or the start of symptoms. Some of my patients have described a psychologically or physically stressful life event around the time the symptoms started, such as a divorce or a car accident. Although this has been some people's experience, the research does not show a direct link between trauma and the onset of MS.

MS is so much more than a scientific definition. It is a journey that comes with uncertainty and fear of disability, but can also lead to determination to live life to the fullest. There is grief from losing function and having life as you knew it change, but it can also open your eyes to new possibilities in the process of adjusting to a "new normal." It is a disease that affects not only the person diagnosed, but also their family and their support community. Proper education and communication is thus a key part of effectively combatting this disease.

CHAPTER 2

....

HOW IS MS DIAGNOSED?

MS is diagnosed based on symptoms and on other clinical evidence. Diagnosis can be challenging both because there is no single test to diagnose the disease and because everyone with MS is unique. Each test or portion of the evaluation serves to gather evidence to determine if the abnormal symptoms or MRIs are likely to be related to demyelination or to some other condition. We want to rule out other reasonable causes for the symptoms, such as other autoimmune diseases, vitamin deficiencies, or infections. Symptoms alone or abnormal tests alone do not equal a diagnosis. If you gather a roomful of people with MS, no two people have exactly the same journey, but there are some symptoms that commonly send people to a neurologist for evaluation. Some wake up with numbness in an arm or leg. Others may see a "spot" in their vision that progresses to visual loss. The symptoms can start suddenly and can worsen over several days.

The first step to diagnosis is a medical history. When you see the neurologist, they will ask questions about the symptoms that brought you into their office and about past symptoms that may have been related to MS. Sometimes, an MS diagnosis may be delayed. This is due to the fact that some symptoms, like leg numbness, could be attributed to a more common diagnosis. For example, a patient with leg numbness may see a doctor who does an x-ray showing arthritis and be diagnosed with a "pinched nerve." The symptoms go away and the patient may never seek further care until something else happens, thereby delaying a diagnosis of possible MS. Symptoms of MS are *very* common to other diseases, and in a young, healthy person, MS may not be at the top of the list for some doctors to investigate. Recent research suggests that risk for MS is increased in African Americans in the US, but overall, MS is not as common in under-represented minorities. Again, this may lead to diagnosis delay if the evaluating physician has a low suspicion.

When evaluating someone for MS, I always ask if my patients remember any past episodes of symptoms that they may have "blown off" or that went away on their own. It is surprising how many people say, "Now that I think about it, a few years ago my leg was numb for a few weeks and it just went away," or, "After I had my baby, I had a little weakness in my arm, but it went away after a while, so I didn't go to the doctor." Those symptoms were possibly the first signs of MS that went unrecognized.

The next part of the evaluation, after the medical history, is the physical exam, most importantly the neurological portion. Believe it or not, there *is* a reason the neurologist makes you touch your nose and then touch their finger. We also don't want to check your reflexes just to see if they are so strong that you kick us (and trust me, I have been kicked a few times). Each part of the neurological exam gives us information about parts of the nervous system that may or may not have been damaged by MS. We look at eye movements, strength, sensation, and coordination, just to name a few things. We can sometimes also see more subtle "signs" of damage that you may not have been aware of, mostly because people don't go around sticking themselves with pins or walking in a straight line on a daily basis.

Something to keep in mind is that although your doctor may find signs of previous nerve damage that is consistent with MS, there are also many who are newly diagnosed that have a completely normal neurological exam. This is often the case after the first relapse, when symptoms commonly resolve themselves. There are other doctors who may see you and think your symptoms are related to MS, but it is important to have the diagnosis confirmed by a neurologist.

Now that you have gotten through the history and physical in the hospital or doctor's office, what happens next? We said that symptoms alone do not make a diagnosis, so there must be other tests that can give us more information, right? Well, I'm so glad you asked, because there is one very important test that can lead to a diagnosis: Magnetic Resonance Imaging (MRI). Prior to the availability of MRI, we used CT scans to diagnose brain and spine conditions. CT scan are helpful in the diagnosis of stroke and acute bleeding in the brain, but not so good at showing the white spots related to MS, especially early on in the disease when there are usually fewer spots present. The development of MRI revolutionized the ability to accurately diagnose MS by showing very detailed images of the brain. Different pictures or "sequences" on an MRI provide information that helps to characterize abnormal areas or spots that are seen in the brain and spine. When we review these images, we look for "white matter lesions" or white spots in areas that are typical of MS. It is important to note that not all white spots equal MS spots. The only way to tell what a spot is with absolute certainty is to do a biopsy, but we certainly don't want to do something that invasive on a regular basis. There are cases where MS lesions look like tumors and do lead to a brain biopsy, but this is rare. Instead, we typically rely on the *size* and *location* of the lesions to help determine what may be causing them. Demyelinating lesions related to MS are usually right next to the fluid-filled areas in the brain called ventricles. White matter lesions in other areas can be related to other conditions, such as migraines, strokes, tumors, or chronic blood vessel damage from diabetes, hypertension, or smoking. Just remember that it is important to discuss your diagnosis with your doctor, because every case of MS is different, and some cases don't fit the "textbook" definition.

There are some people who may not be able to have an MRI because they have a device in their body such as a pacemaker or pain stimulator that would interfere with imaging. An MRI involves a magnet, and we don't want to disrupt or affect metal that is implanted in the body. Diagnosing MS can be very difficult in such cases, and all other information has to be reviewed by a neurologist or possibly an MS specialist to confirm diagnosis. I have also seen people with many different symptoms that suggest MS, but their MRIs are normal. They want to know if it's possible to have MS without having lesions show up on their MRI. The answer is yes and no. Sometimes we may see people very early in the course of the disease before they develop spots. In those cases, we may follow them over time, continue to repeat MRIs, and start treatment once we see the lesions.

There are also cases where someone has a brain MRI for some other reason, like following an accident or for a headache, and there are lesions that look like MS, but the patient may not have noticed symptoms. This is another case that may be followed and monitored by your neurologist over time before deciding to start treatment. Again, it is important to discuss your diagnosis with your doctor, but most of the time a diagnosis is associated with having both lesions appearing on an MRI and neurological symptoms.

MRI results can also be ambiguous or unclear. For instance, an MRI can show white matter lesions that aren't in typical places for MS or don't match with the symptoms reported to the doctor. In these cases, a test called a lumbar puncture, commonly known as a spinal tap, can be performed. Whenever I see a new patient, I ask them if they have had a spinal tap. If they cannot remember, then I know that they definitely *didn't* have one, because a spinal tap is not something people usually forget. A spinal tap is similar to having an epidural, for those who have had babies or who have had the procedure for back pain. The difference is that instead of inserting medicine to numb an area, spinal fluid is removed and sent to a lab for analysis. When we do a spinal tap, we look for antibodies and signs of an overactive immune system. We particularly look for oligoclonal bands, which are found in the spinal fluid of over 80 percent of people with MS. Even with this information, a positive spinal tap alone does not diagnose MS, and, inversely, MS can still exist with the results of a negative test.

Another test to help diagnose MS is called a Visual Evoked Potential (VEP). It is a noninvasive test that is usually done as an outpatient procedure and involves looking at a sequence of visual images in a checkerboard pattern. There are painless wires placed on the scalp, which can record the electrical signals sent to the brain when you see the images; this is used to determine if the signal is recording normally or if it is slowed down due to previous damage to the optic nerve. In some cases, this type of test can also be done while testing auditory and sensory functions. This can tell us if there are subtle changes related to previous demyelination. VEP testing usually shows abnormal results in people who have had optic neuritis, but can be abnormal even if you don't recall having visual loss related to MS.

During an evaluation for MS, we also look for or "rule out" other conditions that can mimic the neurological symptoms or lesions seen with MS. For example, a panel of bloodwork is done to screen for other diseases that can mimic MS, including vitamin deficiencies, rheumatologic diseases like lupus, and infectious diseases like Lyme disease. When a spinal tap is done, we can also look at other things in the spinal fluid, like indicators for Lyme disease or other infections or for signs of cancer cells.

MS diagnosis is not always easy. I jokingly tell some of my patients that they forgot to read the textbook before they came in to see me. It may take a while, but it is important not to be too hasty in making a diagnosis, as it essentially commits a person to a lifetime of treatment that can affect the immune system and may have long-term consequences. Sometimes the diagnosis takes time, and you may have to have several MRIs before it's confirmed. If you have been diagnosed, it's important to keep following up with your neurologist so that they can make adjustments to your treatment as needed.

CHAPTER 3

··

WHAT TYPE OF MS DO I HAVE? HOW CAN I PLAN FOR MY FUTURE?

One of the biggest challenges of MS is the uncertainty about the future. Symptoms often start in people ages twenty through forty, a period of time which is full of significant life planning. You might be in college or graduate school, starting a new career, planning a family, or in the middle of raising children. Then the MS diagnosis comes and turns everything upside down.

"What type of MS do I have?" is a common question after receiving a diagnosis. We currently use several terms to categorize MS, including relapsing-remitting, primary progressive, and secondary progressive. It is thought that 85 percent of people are initially diagnosed with a "relapsing-remitting" disease, and at least 50 percent go on to develop "secondary progressive disease." Only about 10–15 percent of people are initially diagnosed with primary progressive disease. As our understanding of MS continues to evolve, many in the scientific community are trying to find more accurate ways to describe the disease. For example, we now recognize that relapses and progression can be happening simultaneously. Although the categories are not perfect, they are the best we have.

To discuss relapsing-remitting disease, we must first define a relapse. An MS exacerbation, or relapse, is an episode of new symptoms or the worsening of old ones that lasts from several days to weeks. The period following a relapse, during which symptoms stabilize or go away, is called a remission. It is important to note that remissions with MS are not the same as cancer remissions. With cancer remission, we cannot find evidence of the disease in the body. An MS remission does not mean that the disease is completely quiet. A person can feel well, but still have new lesions forming in the brain and spine. Also, not all relapses result in complete recovery, so a remission could represent a stable level of disability. For instance, if you have a relapse causing numbness in your leg and the symptoms get 90 percent better, then it stays that way for six months, we would call that a remission.

Other categories associated with MS include clinically isolated syndrome and radiographically isolated syndrome. When a person has one episode of symptoms typical of MS and an MRI that shows a lesion in a place specific for demyelination, it is called clinically isolated syndrome. People who fit in this category are treated for MS because they have a very high risk of going on to develop further symptoms of MS. A radiographically isolated syndrome occurs when an MRI is done for some other reason, such as a car accident or a headache, and the MRI looks very typical of MS, but the person has not had symptoms of MS. In such a case, most people follow up with a neurologist with repeat MRIs, and if they have any new neurological symptoms, they will likely start treatment.

Other forms of MS can be progressive. As stated earlier, about 10 to 15 percent of people diagnosed will have primary progressive MS. This means that once the symptoms start, they continually worsen. So, instead of the disease being characterized by symptoms that come and go suddenly, patients notice that things just get worse over time. Another form of MS is secondary progressive. This means that a person started off with relapsing-remitting disease, and over time, usually over ten to twenty years, they begin to notice worsening instead of relapses. For example, I've had patients say, "Dr. Williams, last spring I was able to walk two miles with my dog, but this year, I can only walk one mile." The progression is often slow and sometimes may also be noticed by family members and friends. Although these are the common categories we use to describe MS, they are not perfect. Many times, people may have a bit of both processes going on at the same time. There are efforts to use models that better describe the complex process of MS, but these are the current categories in use.

If symptoms do not completely resolve after the first relapse, many patients question if they will improve and be able to return to work and their regular daily activities. If the symptoms have improved, there may be anxiety about if the symptoms will come back or if something worse will happen. This fear of the future can be paralyzing, especially for those who have minimal or no disability. However, none of us can predict the future. There are some people who start off with very severe symptoms and completely improve, and others who do well at first and then take a turn for the worse. I have seen people improve from using a wheelchair to walking and vice versa.

There are certain characteristics, called prognostic factors, that can help us understand who may have a milder or more difficult journey with their MS. Some good prognostic factors include diagnosis at an older age, having just one symptom at the start of the disease, and having complete recovery between relapses. Poor prognostic factors include a younger diagnosis, having multiple symptoms at the start of the disease, being a man, and being African American. These are all possible predictors, but every person is different, so having poor prognostic factors doesn't automatically mean that you will have an aggressive disease or severe disability from your MS.

The most important thing is to remember that we cross every bridge when we get to it, and some bridges we hopefully will never have to cross. MS can cause disability, but there are many people with MS who are living very full lives, raising families, working, and enjoying life. When people pass away from complications of MS, it is generally for the same reason that people who have any other type of significant physical disability pass away: from some type of infection. I often say, "MS is not a death sentence, but it is an adjustment sentence." We don't want to spend all of our time worrying about things that could happen, because if they don't happen, we worried for nothing. If they do happen, we wasted a lot of good time worrying about it and it happened anyway. However, I also recognize that the fear and uncertainty are very real and difficult to grapple with for many people. I generally recommend building a good support network of family and friends, as well as connecting with other people living with MS who can understand exactly what you are going through. Also, I generally refer to psychological counseling for my newly diagnosed patients, since it can be overwhelming to deal with the diagnosis in addition to all the other general stressors of life.

....

CHAPTER 4

HOW DO YOU TREAT MS?

The treatment of multiple sclerosis has changed tremendously over the past twenty years. MS was recognized as a disease in the late 1800s, but the first FDA approved medication didn't become available until 1993. Before that, some severe cases of MS were treated with chemotherapy drugs, but most people had no treatment at all. Once steroids were known to alleviate symptoms of MS, many people took them to help with the symptoms, but this did not seem to slow the progression of MS or prevent further lesions from showing up on an MRI. Also, chronic steroid use can lead to complications like elevated blood sugar, elevated blood pressure, and osteoporosis. When the initial treatment, Interferon Beta, became available, patients had to enter a lottery to determine who could receive this groundbreaking treatment. The great news is that since 1993, there have been multiple new therapies tested and approved for multiple sclerosis. This is really an exciting time to be in the field of MS, because as we have more options available, we can choose the ones that will best treat people living with this disease. Not only do we have fourteen available therapies for MS at the time I'm writing this book, there are also many exciting new options on the horizon. I am not going to detail specific therapies and side effects in this chapter; instead, I'd like to talk more about the general approach to treatment. It is important to educate yourself about available options and have a discussion with your doctor to determine the best treatment for you.

I like to look at treatment as a four-layer cake, because, well, I like cake! The first layer of the cake is acute treatment. If you call your doctor because you suddenly lost vision in one eye or developed leg weakness, they will usually have you come to the office for an assessment and to discuss treatment for a relapse. The most common treatment for relapse is corticosteroids, which can be given by infusion or by mouth. The steroids are given to help speed up your body's ability to recover. They do not, however, significantly decrease your immune system's attack on your central nervous system over time. We usually give them over a short period of time because chronic steroid use can cause side effects, including swelling, weight gain, and elevated blood sugar. They can also temporarily make you a little more hungry or irritable. Now, if you received a short course of steroids for three days, and four or five months later you are still overeating, that is because you just want to eat—that's not the steroids still working! This is a short-term solution for decreasing inflammation in the nervous system, but is generally not a long-term solution for treating the disease.

Now let's focus for a bit on the second layer of the cake: disease-modifying therapy. These medications help decrease the likelihood that your immune system will attack your myelin in a variety of ways. There are three forms of therapy in this layer: injections, pills, and infusions. One of the unique things about MS therapy is that most of the medications work on different pathways and cells in the immune system to decrease the overall activity. Some can decrease the factors that produce inflammatory immune cells, others may deplete or remove the overactive immune cells, and still others may block the cells from entering the central nervous system space to attack myelin and cause disability. Because they work in different ways, it means they may have different side effects. That is why it's important for you and your doctor to discuss options and side effects—as well as other conditions you have and medications you take that may interfere with some side effects—to determine the best plan for you. As we have more options available, we can usually find a treatment that is both tolerable and effective for your MS.

The third layer of the cake is symptom management. There are many neurological symptoms that can be related to MS. Some people have mostly physical symptoms, like weakness and difficulty walking, while others may have more "silent symptoms" of MS, like cognitive problems and fatigue—which we will discuss in a later chapter. Most often, there will be some combination of both. I do not recommend that anyone memorize a complete list of MS symptoms, because it will scare you to death! It is rare that someone has every possible symptom of MS. It is also important to remember that people with MS can have the same problems that other people have, and that not everything is necessarily the MS. This layer of symptom management is important because this is where we can really make an impact on your daily life. This layer is also what you spend the majority of your time discussing at your doctor visits. There are some symptoms that we can help treat, like numbness and tingling, urinary frequency, and spasticity. There are other symptoms that, unfortunately, we don't have treatments for, like visual loss. I often explain to my patients that there is a part that you play and a part that medication plays. If you have spasticity or cramping, for example, medications can help relax the muscles, but it also helps if you stretch on a regular basis or do exercises like yoga. We also have to carefully balance benefits with side effects, because some of the symptomatic treatments can increase other MS symptoms, like fatigue or cognitive dysfunction.

Finally, the fourth layer of the cake involves therapy. Some people include this in the symptom management category, but I would much rather have four layers in a cake than three! There are several forms of therapy that can benefit people living with MS. I often refer people to physical therapy for problems like weakness, gait imbalance, and spasticity. A physical therapist can help develop an exercise program specific to your needs. They can also help with assessing which assistive device for walking is the best for your needs, whether that's a cane, walker, motorized scooter, or wheelchair. Occupational therapy helps with activities of daily living, like making sure you can feed yourself or button your clothes, especially if you have problems with coordination or numbness in the fingers, which can limit your dexterity. Speech therapy may be needed if you have trouble swallowing or difficulty talking due to slurred speech. Also, cognitive therapy may be helpful for cognitive dysfunction related to MS, such as slowed processing. Finally, vocational rehabilitation can assist with job assessment if disability from MS keeps you from going back to your former job.

Although the cake is a simple way to think of the layers to MS treatment, we can see a few things from this example. One is that there is not just one approach to treating MS, and each treatment plan will be individualized. Another thing to recognize is that there may be a need for readjustment of the plan, so if something is not working, you should have another conversation with your physician about potential ways to adjust the plan as your needs change over time.

CHAPTER 5

THERE'S NO CURE FOR MS, SO WHY SHOULD I START TREATMENT?

When I ask a newly diagnosed person what they know about MS, one of the most common phrases I hear is, "I know that there's no cure." While this is true, if we look at things in a broader context, most chronic diseases in medicine are managed, and there are very few that we can actually cure. Think about common diseases like hypertension, diabetes, or thyroid disease. These conditions are treated and monitored by your doctor over time. Part of the reason this phrase is problematic is because it can cause a sense of hopelessness. The immune system is a complex system, with many different cells and pathways involved. The more we learn, the more we seek different approaches to attack this potentially debilitating disease. One thing we have learned is that it's important to start treatment as early as possible to try to prevent long-term disability. The body can heal itself to a certain extent, but it takes time to see how close someone will return to normal after the start of MS symptoms, and each relapse has the potential to cause disability. The real goal is to keep you living life to the fullest and achieving as much as possible with MS.

There are three goals that we have in mind when starting disease-modifying therapy. The goals of therapy are to decrease the risk of having a relapse, to decrease the risk of forming new white matter lesions on your MRI, and to slow down the progression of the disease. Unfortunately, we don't have medicines that fix the damage that's already been done to the nervous system; our current treatments try to prevent new damage. In other words, we can't fix what's already broken, but we do try to prevent new things from being broken.

So how do we know if it's working? If you feel the same and your MRIs look the same. I spend a lot of time setting treatment goals with my patients, because it is important that we are on the same page with our expectations. Most of the time, when we take medicine for a symptom or condition, we expect the condition to get better, but this generally is not the case with MS therapy, and this needs to be clearly explained at the time of treatment initiation. If you feel better or notice an improvement, it is more likely to be your body healing itself slowly over time. There are some people who report feeling better on just about all of the current MS treatments, but this is not what the medications are formulated to do. I tell my patients that my ultimate goal is to have "social visits" with them, where we talk mostly about vacations and they show me family pictures, because their MS is stable. There are some drugs that may be considered more effective than others, but since everyone's MS is different, you could potentially be on a "less effective" drug, but have it work very well to treat your MS.

We live in an age that is focusing more and more on holistic health. People are trying different diets and forms of exercise to improve their overall health. As a result, I have some people who ask about having dieting and exercise be the only intervention to treat their MS. A healthy, well-balanced diet and physical activity will definitely improve health for a person with a chronic disease like MS. However, these interventions alone do not modify the overactivity of the immune system. Most of my patients who choose this option come back because of worsening or new symptoms. The fundamental problem with this approach is that once the damage has been done, we can't go back and fix it. The earlier we start with therapy, the better chance we have of preventing disability. Another challenge of MS is that the disease can sometimes be "quiet" physically for years, but just because you don't feel anything, that doesn't mean that the MS isn't causing more damage. New lesions can form in the brain without symptoms and may cause disability later on in life.

There are some people who just don't want to start treatment. Maybe it's denial of the diagnosis, fear of medication side effects, or dislike of the idea of putting foreign substances into their bodies. These are all valid concerns, and are issues that I address on a regular basis. I see many patterns in this disease, and as we have discussed, there's no way to reliably predict the course of MS. I do have an occasional patient who did not go on therapy and appeared to do well for some time, but this is a very small minority of patients that I've seen during my career. Most of the time, there is either a relapse or a subsequent MRI showing increased lesions, which leads to another conversation about treatment. Unfortunately, I have seen many who stop going to the doctor altogether and get much worse before they come back to be treated.

Although there are many concerns about starting treatment, most often treatment does make a difference! It's true that it is not perfect and there are side effects.

Some people may be anxious enough about listed side effects that they don't want to start treatment at all. But remember: all the side effects that you get warnings about are only potential side effects. There are many people that do well and tolerate therapy well. If you are having side effects, let your doctor know so that you can discuss other options. I will repeat this because it is really important. While there are some rare exceptions, with the options we have available we can find a DMT, a disease-modifying therapy, that will treat your MS with side effects that you can tolerate. Regardless of your decision about therapy, it's important to keep checking in with your doctor for physical exams and repeat MRIs to see if there are any changes. Also, make sure that you commit to whatever regimen you and your doctor discuss. There is no treatment that completely gets rid of all MS symptoms, but if you are taking your medicine regularly and your MS is getting worse, we need to know it's because your medicine isn't working, not because you're not taking it.

Just like it's important to know when to start treatment, it is also important to know when to stop treatment. There are a few reasons for discontinuing therapy. If you continue to have relapses despite taking your medication, it may mean that it is not working well enough. If you or your family feel that you are continuing to worsen despite treatment, that is another reason to address your therapy. If your MRIs continue to show new lesions, it can also mean your DMT is not working, and you need to switch to a different treatment. MRIs give us a "sneak peek" at what is going on under the surface in your brain and allow us to intervene and in many cases change course before we see physical symptoms. Although most of our current therapies are approved for relapsing MS, you and your doctor may feel that another option would provide additional benefits. Finally, if you cannot tolerate your medications or if the side effects are interfering with your daily life, talk to your doctor about other options.

CHAPTER 6

BUT YOU LOOK SO GOOD; HOW CAN YOU HAVE MS?

As I mentioned earlier, one reason that diagnosing MS can be difficult is because the symptoms are very similar to symptoms of common diseases. Numbness and tingling in an arm can be related to other conditions, like a pinched nerve or carpal tunnel syndrome. Dizziness can be related to an inner ear infection. So if a young, healthy person comes in with mild symptoms, it may be diagnosed as a common condition. The good news is that the treatment for many of these symptoms is the same, whether it is caused by MS or by other conditions. It is not uncommon that when people come to me for diagnosis, they are already on appropriate symptomatic therapy.

We must also keep in mind that each additional medication has potential side effects, so we have to balance the risks and benefits. For instance, many of our symptomatic medications can cause sedation, which can worsen fatigue. It's almost like walking a tightrope, because the solution to one problem can worsen another.

Physical symptoms like weakness or difficulty walking are easy for people to grasp and associate with disability. It is more difficult, however, to understand the invisible or silent symptoms of MS that can cause significant disability. One of the things I frequently hear from my patients is that people tell them, "You look so good, I didn't know you have MS," or, "You don't look sick." They also may get nasty looks when they park in a handicapped parking spot, even though muscle fatigue related to walking long distances can make it hard to get to the car after a shopping trip. Family members or friends of my patients may think that they are being lazy when they say they have fatigue, or may mistake cognitive dysfunction for them ignoring conversations. In this chapter, I'd like to focus on some of these silent symptoms that interrupt daily life.

Let's start with fatigue. This is a very common symptom of MS that can be debilitating and lead to leaving the workforce. It is not your run-of-the-mill tired feeling after a long day of work. For instance, my current routine after a long day of work, with a husband and two young children, is to come home, make dinner, play with my daughter, do homework with my son, bathe the kids, and get them ready for bed. Then I fix lunch for the kindergartener, fix my own lunch, shower, and chat with my hubby before getting on the computer to finish working on this book! I know about being tired, but I recognize that the fatigue my patients describe is very different from what I experience after a long day of being a doctor, mommy, and wife.

MS fatigue is a distinct entity that is well recognized in the field. Most people describe it like they "run out of gas" or "hit a brick wall." I had one person describe it as a heaviness, like "walking underwater with a fur coat on." There's a finite amount of energy for the day, and when you get up in the morning, you have to be careful of how you use it. If you do too much, it can be completely gone by noon; or, if you pace yourself, you may be able to make it through the workday, but when you get home, you "crash" and have to go to bed. The fatigue can be so disabling that it can actually lead to filing for disability from work. It usually worsens as the day progresses. Sometimes if you take a rest (like a power nap) during the day, it can be like a "reset" and you get more energy. However, this is not feasible for everyone, especially if they work full time. Also, there are other causes of fatigue that may add on to the MS fatigue, making it much more severe. For example, insomnia, depression, and some medications can cause fatigue as well. Make sure that you are working with your doctor to identify the contributors to your fatigue and create a plan to treat it.

The first step in developing an action plan is to determine the contributors to your fatigue, because often MS itself may cause a small portion of the fatigue, but other factors are worsening the symptom to the point that it interferes with your daily life. Sleep disturbance is a common cause of increased fatigue. Insomnia can be related to depression or anxiety, or to other MS symptoms, like pain or frequent urination. Also, many of us generally have poor sleep hygiene, meaning we do everything in bed but sleep. We read on our tablets, play on social media, or watch television. Over time, our bodies don't associate the bed with sleep, which makes it hard to sleep well. Additionally, diet and exercise affect our energy levels, so eating a healthy, well-balanced diet and doing light exercise several days a week can have a large impact on this symptom. If you have severe fatigue, your doctor may recommend that you use stimulants.

Energy conservation is a subject I frequently counsel my patients about. It is very hard to transition from life before MS to life after MS if fatigue is a major factor. If you are used to functioning at a certain level and being able to go constantly, it can be challenging to adjust to a new normal. You can still try to do everything, but you often wind up paying for it because it takes your body longer to recover. So you may do a ton of activities one day, but then you're worn out and extremely tired for two or three days after that. Having a good day followed by two bad days does not lead to a good quality of life. The goal is to spread out activities so that you can be active to some degree on a daily basis. It's difficult to find that balance, but it is possible. Keys to finding this balance include learning to say "no" to unnecessary activities, delegating tasks to others, and leaning on your support network and partners in care for help.

Another silent and often embarrassing symptom of MS is bladder dysfunction. This problem is a bit more common among people with forms of MS that include spinal cord involvement. It is not something that other people can see, but it can be not only mentally distressing, but also extremely disruptive to daily routines. I like to classify bladder problems into two simple categories: "gotta go, gotta go, gotta go," or "gotta go and can't go." Some people have urinary "frequency," meaning you have to go to the restroom often throughout the day. They may also have "urgency," which means you get the urge to urinate, then, if you don't get to the bathroom fast, you could actually have incontinence or an accident. This is very embarrassing for many people, especially if they have ever had an unexpected episode of incontinence in public and had to find a way to clean up and change clothes. It is also difficult to deal with wearing pads or protective undergarments, especially for young women. In severe cases, I've seen some people limit their activities and avoid places that may not have easily accessible restrooms. In cases of retention (or gotta go and can't go), people feel like they have to urinate, but there may be a delay for the urine to come out. This can potentially lead to frequent bladder infections.

Identifying and addressing other factors that cause bladder dysfunction is key to treatment. Urinary tract infections can cause temporary changes in bladder function; you should be tested if you have a sudden change or worsening in bladder function. In women, changes to the pelvic structures after having babies can cause bladder dysfunction. A consultation with an OB-GYN may help determine a course of treatment. In men, prostate enlargement can affect urination. Again, it's important to rule out other causes before we attribute a symptom to the MS. There are medications that can treat urinary frequency and retention. Other treatments include use of a catheter to empty the bladder or botulinum toxin

(Botox) injections in the bladder. These treatments require a referral to a urologist, a specialist that deals with bladder dysfunction.

Cognitive dysfunction is an under-recognized silent symptom of MS. It is also a major reason why people leave the workforce and apply for long-term disability. The signs can be subtle at first. Maybe you have a little trouble finding words while talking to someone, or you frequently lose your train of thought. Family members and friends may tell you that your memory is bad, that you ask the same questions over and over, or that you completely forgot a recent conversation. If they are not aware that this is a symptom related to MS, they may mistakenly think you are ignoring them, not listening, or not paying attention. One of the best ways to deal with cognitive dysfunction is education, especially of family and friends. The most common cognitive problems with MS are slowed processing of information, easy distractibility, and impaired attention and concentration. When you add all these things together, it equals a short-term memory problem. Just like many other silent symptoms, there are other conditions that can affect cognition, too. Fatigue and depression can affect your thinking in ways similar to MS. Very often, MS is playing a part in the problem, but when you add the other conditions on top of it, the symptom becomes so severe that it interferes with your ability to function at home and at work.

Treatment involves several approaches. Your doctor may refer you for neuropsychological testing to evaluate your memory and thinking problems. The testing takes most of a day and involves an interview and written portions. It helps to determine the severity of cognition changes due to MS and what other factors, like depression, may be involved. There are no specific medications that treat cognitive function, but you should work with your doctor to determine if your disease-modifying therapy is working for you or if interventions like cognitive therapy may be appropriate.

CHAPTER 7

. . . .

SAY WHAT? I DIDN'T KNOW BLACK PEOPLE GOT MS!

MS has been recognized as a disease that occurs mostly in young Caucasian women. Although globally this is still the most common group to have MS, the scientific community is beginning to understand how the disease may look different in different populations. In the US, we are learning more about MS in ethnic minority populations, specifically African Americans. Several studies published in 2012 and 2013 suggested that the risk for MS in the US may be highest in African Americans. This is quite shocking, because it was traditionally thought that African Americans were not commonly affected by MS. It is now becoming recognized that not only does MS occur more frequently than we thought in people of African descent, but the disease also may behave differently in this population.

Out of over 60,000 articles about MS in medical journals, only a little over one hundred articles have been published about MS in ethnic minority populations in the US, and they primarily describe the disease in African American and Latino populations. Most of these studies look at populations retrospectively, meaning we have a group of people and we look back and see how they did, then describe it. Although this is good research, a better way to look at disease is prospectively, meaning we start with a group of people that are on a "level playing field" and look forward to see how they will perform under the same circumstances and given the same treatment. This type of research can give us an idea of barriers that may make one group do worse, long term, than another one.

Over the past ten years, I have had many African Americans sit in my office and say, "Dr. Mitzi, no one in my family has MS and I don't even know anybody with MS who looks like me. How did I get this disease?" Frankly, until the past ten or fifteen years, MS was not a diagnosis on the top of the list for young African Americans with neurological symptoms, and not much was known about the disease in this group. There are many possible reasons for this, including disparities in socioeconomic status and access to care. Also, as imaging tests such as MRIs became much more accessible in the past ten years, the diagnosis has become easier to make.

Although the amount of research is small, there are some trends that we see from the information available. The most striking data shows trends suggesting that African Americans may have a more "aggressive" course of disease compared to other ethnic groups. There may be more lesions in the spinal cord, more visual difficulty at the time of diagnosis, and a greater subsequent disability over time. Some studies suggest that walking disabilities occur earlier in the disease for African Americans and that the time to needing a walking assistive device such as a cane can be eight to ten years earlier than Caucasians with MS. MRI studies suggest that African Americans have more severe white matter lesions with less myelin repair. At diagnosis, there may be a more "vigorous" immune response, with higher numbers of oligoclonal bands in the spinal fluid. There are also some suggestions that the response to treatments may be different in different populations.

We don't know why we see these differences. Limited studies on access to care observed that African Americans are less likely to be cared for by a neurologist, which means they may be less likely to have a treatment plan and adequate treatment of symptoms. Socioeconomic status may affect access to care or specialty centers. It may also affect access to starting and staying on medication. Or, resources may be unrecognized and thus unused in the African American community. There have been some genetic differences identified, but it is unclear what role they play and if that is really the driving force for the clinical differences we see.

Every week I see several newly diagnosed African Americans with MS. It is disheartening to see the level of disability some people have so early after diagnosis. There are many questions that are unanswered, and there is a great deal of work to be done to better understand this disease. This lack of knowledge is partially because the research studies that inform the way we understand and treat disease are done in mostly European populations, with very little enrollment of ethnic minority populations. Ideally, we want our research to reflect what we see in the real world, including the variety of people in the studies.

Limited studies in Latino populations reveal that an MS diagnosis tends to occur earlier in life and there are some differences in the way the spinal cord lesions look on MRI. There is some data available about MS in other ethnic minority groups, including Asian populations, and there may be some similar characteristics to African Americans. Ultimately, though, more research is needed.

CHAPTER 8

··

WHY SHOULD I
PARTICIPATE IN RESEARCH?

Before medications are approved to be tested in humans, they are usually tested in animal models of a disease to understand how the medicines work and to identify potential side effects. If a medicine seems to work in the animal model of the disease, and the potential benefits seem to outweigh the side effects, then it may be approved for human testing. There are ethics committees that must approve studies that are done in humans, so there are very strict standards to ensure that people are not abused or mistreated during research. In fact, the care provided for people in research trials is not only very good, it is also often free. Doctor visits, imaging, and medications are covered, and if a person continues on therapy after the trial is finished, they may be eligible to continue in the "extension phase" of the research.

When we think of clinical research, a common type of study that comes to mind is a large clinical trial. Clinical trials for MS are often conducted with patients and physicians across the globe and lead to approval of medications or medical procedures. They have strict criteria for who can and can't participate in the study and have well-documented requirements and protocols. There are generally limits on age (between ages eighteen to fifty-five) and criteria for disease activity and level of disability when entering the trial. This is an attempt to "level the playing field" and make sure that changes in condition are due to MS and treatment effects as opposed to other things. Everyone starts out with similar characteristics and receives similar care so we can see how they do over time.

Although there are many benefits to this type of research, there are some drawbacks. For example, strict criteria may also exclude people of different ages and with other medical conditions that may interfere with the medications involved, but which occur commonly in the real world in people who need to be treated. In addition, restrictions on the level of disability may leave out people who have had MS for a long time or who have significant disability.

There are four phases of clinical trials:

- Phase 1 trials are usually conducted with small numbers of people to make sure that medications are safe to proceed with in further trials in human models.

- Phase 2 trials are conducted in slightly larger numbers of people. These trials also monitor side effects, but primarily try to determine if the medication is effective in treating the disease state.

- Phase 3 trials are conducted in many clinics and sites in different parts of the world. They usually involve larger numbers of people, and they try to determine the effectiveness of the medication and any common side effects or other, potentially serious side effects. For most MS medications, at least two large Phase 3 trials are needed for drug approval, but in some cases it could be more or less than that.

- Phase 4 trials are done after a medication is approved and already on the market. These trials usually look at different issues, such as tolerability, quality of life measures, and patient satisfaction with therapy.

Safety and side effects are important and monitored even after medications are approved. Research trials are very carefully conducted, but sometimes other issues will arise after a medication is out in the "real world" with a large number of people taking it. The FDA is continually updated about side effects, and the medication information is updated if new issues become apparent. In some cases, a medication can be withdrawn from the market if unforeseen side effects are severe. It may also happen that side effects that seemed very common in a trial may not be as common as we thought after it gets out into the real world.

Although very important, clinical trials are only one form of research. Research can involve questionnaires, surveys, and other interventions. Registries collect basic information and follow up with questions over time. There are also studies that measure the effects of interventions like exercise programs or diet changes to improve quality of life. There are many different ways to contribute to the increasing knowledge about MS and help everyone living with this disease.

Research informs how we treat medical conditions. Why is it important to participate in research? Because we all need to stand up and be counted. If only one group of people participates in the research, how do we know that the results apply to everyone? We may be missing unique cultural and genetic differences that can help us treat the disease more accurately, or we may even be missing the key to a cure! Clinical trials are not for everyone, but there is SOME way that everyone can be involved. Whether it's a registry, a questionnaire, or a survey, get in where you fit in! I encourage all of my patients to participate in research so we can continue to learn and grow as an MS community.

. . . .

CHAPTER 9

WHY IS THERE SO LITTLE DIVERSITY IN RESEARCH?

Most of the advances that we make in medicine are tied to research. That research comes in a variety of forms, but as I mentioned earlier, we learn a great deal of information from clinical trials. These large studies are controlled and enroll people with similar characteristics, who then receive the same level of care so we are able to measure treatment outcomes. There are several groups that are frequently underrepresented in our MS research, including ethnic minorities and people over the age of fifty-five.

The history of research in the minority community has been difficult, especially for African Americans in the US. There have been many injustices, ranging from unwilling experimentation on slaves to the Tuskegee syphilis study, which withheld curative treatment for syphilis once it became available in order to observe the end stages of the disease. Interactions with the medical system have been fraught with experiences of discrimination and bias, leading to many of the disparities and inequities we see in medical care today. This has led some to mistrust the healthcare system, including the motives of healthcare research. Fortunately, research trial protocols are now rigorously reviewed to ensure that human rights are not violated and that the work done is ethical. These protections are for all people, and try to ensure that everyone gets equal care and no one is taken advantage of.

Despite the history of mistreatment, it seems that there is an increasing willingness in people from ethnic minority groups to participate in clinical research. Surveys and polls suggest that although African Americans may report having experienced discrimination in the healthcare system, they actually want to be involved in research studies. Some of the motivation is to help others in their community who may suffer from the same conditions. Barriers to participation include difficulty finding information about research in their area or not being asked by their doctor to participate. There is very little research on MS in diverse communities as compared to the overall body of literature about MS. When we look at the large research studies, although it is estimated that 10–30 percent of the US MS population is African American, our research studies average less than 5 percent enrollment in clinical trials.

Another population that is often overlooked is people over the age of fifty-five. Most of our trials enroll people between the ages of eighteen and fifty-five, but there is a growing population of people living with MS who don't fit in this range, which presents new challenges to treatment. Just as our bodies change as we get older, our immune systems also change as we age. There are some who believe that MS generally "burns out" or becomes inactive after a certain age, but, as with so many aspects of MS, everyone is different. We need to better understand the effects of treatment over time, and study if our therapies may interact with the aging immune system to cause higher risk for certain side effects over time. It is not clear if people should be taken off therapy just because of their age, and we need more evidence to support the best way to treat this population.

As scientific knowledge continues to evolve, the medical community is constantly looking for better ways to manage medical conditions. We want to move toward finding ways to determine the best treatment for an individual. Scientists are looking for "markers" to see if we can predict how someone responds to treatment. The goal is to be able to look at a person who is diagnosed with a certain disease and pick a treatment based on their individual makeup. This type of treatment paradigm is called "personalized medicine." But if a limited group of people engage in the research, it may be difficult to generalize the results for everyone else.

It is not necessarily easy to find ways to participate in research independently. There are websites of MS charitable organizations that may detail research studies that are being conducted in your area or that are funded by the organization. You can ask your doctor if their practice is participating in any research activities and if you qualify for them. You can also ask if there are other clinics or facilities locally that participate in research. Finally, you can look at academic or teaching hospitals in the area and contact their research departments to see if there are studies available.

It is also important for health care providers to develop a trusting relationship with their patients to facilitate communication and improve willingness to take advice and suggestions. Patients can be leery of motives if they don't trust their doctor. There can also be unconscious bias on the part of the physicians. They may have perceptions of certain groups of people based on previous experience. These are things that definitely need to be addressed in the healthcare field, and I am fortunate to be working on several projects to increase education for patients and providers about the need for increased diversity in clinical research.

CHAPTER 10

....

SO WHAT CAN I DO TO HELP MYSELF?

First, let's say this: there is nothing that you did physically to cause MS, and there is nothing you can do to make it worse, except stopping whatever treatment plan you and your doctor choose without consulting your neurologist. Even though the disease can worsen unexpectedly, there are still things you can do to improve your overall health and live well with MS. I will say it again, there is a part you play and a part the medication plays. There is no medication that will do everything for you or erase what you can do to improve your own health.

One thing that you can do to live better with MS is to eat a healthy, well-balanced diet. Many people ask me if there are certain foods they should eat or avoid. It is always helpful to consult a dietician or nutritionist about specific dietary plans. There is not one specific diet that makes MS better or worse, but a healthy diet can improve health outcomes for anyone, especially someone living with a chronic disease like MS. I have patients who have been on every type of diet imaginable, including variations of gluten-free, paleo, and vegan regimens. Some people need strict requirements to maintain a healthy lifestyle and others can just make adjustments on their own. Many of these plans incorporate more raw and fresh foods and less processed foods. Although it is important to read labels to know what's in your food, my mantra is, most of the time, when we put it in our mouths, we know if we should be eating it or not. Additional benefits of a healthy diet are possible improvements in fatigue and constipation.

Exercise can provide many benefits for people living with MS, such as helping with muscle weakness, fatigue, spasticity, and constipation. Physical activity can also be a mood booster and a stress reducer for those struggling with depression and anxiety. Sometimes it's hard to know where to get started, so you should consult your doctor before starting any exercise plan. I often recommend reframing our thoughts about exercise as well. When we think of working out, a mental image of someone with a fashionable outfit accompanied by washboard abs exercising at the gym for an hour may come to mind. That may not be the case for you, depending on how you are affected by MS. The goal is to move more; that may be fifteen or twenty minutes of walking, swimming, or doing yoga a few days a week. You should start off slow and advance your activity at your own pace. It may be helpful to start with a referral to physical therapy. A physiatrist or physical therapist can help assess your strengths and form a targeted exercise program focused on your specific issues. They can also provide recommendations if you need a device or brace to help with walking, such as a cane, a walker, or an AFO brace to help with foot drop. Whatever your approach, remember to listen to your body. Rest if you need to and know that overdoing it could result in you feeling poorly for a few days afterward.

Stress management is another key component to managing symptoms of MS. Many wonder if stress can bring on relapses. There has been limited research done, and there is no clear link between stress and relapses. However, there does appear to be a connection between stress and pseudo-relapses. A pseudo-relapse is a temporary worsening of symptoms related to conditions such as heat exposure and infection. Many of my patients feel that their symptoms are worsened with stress. It affects their ability to function in daily activities, such as work and family duties, and can take a toll on the body if not adequately treated. It's important to find positive outlets to deal with stress effectively. These can include spending time with family and friends (only if they don't make you more stressed out!), doing something you enjoy, or exercising. It is also important to note that sometimes people use the word "stress," but they really have symptoms of depression or anxiety. It is important to have this assessed and treated properly. I also encourage you to obtain support from like-minded people with MS, because it is important to engage with others who truly understand what you are facing.

Another thing you can do is to stop smoking cigarettes if you are still doing so, because smoking can negatively impact the course of your disease and possibly worsen relapses. Newer research also suggests that obesity may worsen MS as well. This is not an exhaustive list of lifestyle changes to help people living with MS, but it is a great place to start.

YOU are your own best advocate! Make sure that you educate yourself about your condition and understand what your treatments are supposed to do. Attend programs to learn more about options as they become available. Look for reliable sources of information and continue to learn. Know your body and keep track of your symptoms. Make sure that you let your doctor know if you are having issues with your medications or difficulty taking them. That way, if you're having problems, they know it is because the medication is not working, and not because you are not taking it. Involve family and friends in the process. They may be able to see or recognize any worsening of symptoms or remember details that you don't recall. Although a diagnosis of MS can be life changing, you can live well with MS. Living well may look different for each person, but with the support of your loved ones and your healthcare team, it is possible to achieve this goal.

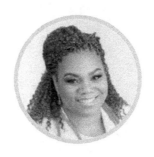

ABOUT THE AUTHOR

Dr. Mitzi Williams is a board-certified neurologist and multiple sclerosis specialist. She has presented research both nationally and internationally about MS in diverse populations and is sought after as a speaker and consultant. She also works on several national steering committees focused on increasing diversity in clinical trials and addressing disparities in ethnic minority populations with MS.

Dr. Mitzi sees it as her mission to engage, educate, and empower people affected by MS so they can become an active part of their healthcare teams, as well as to increase diversity in clinical research. She is passionate about serving others and about her faith, her family, and education, and in her free time she enjoys singing, reading, and attending concerts and plays. Dr. Mitzi lives in Atlanta with her husband, Bernard, and their two children.

To connect, email her at info@drmitzijoimd.com

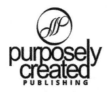

CREATING DISTINCTIVE BOOKS
WITH INTENTIONAL RESULTS

We're a collaborative group of creative masterminds
with a mission to produce high-quality books to position
you for monumental success in the marketplace.

Our professional team of writers, editors, designers,
and marketing strategists work closely together to ensure
that every detail of your book is a clear representation
of the message in your writing.

Want to know more?
Write to us at info@publishyourgift.com
or call (888) 949-6228

Discover great books, exclusive offers, and more at
www.PublishYourGift.com

Connect with us on social media

@publishyourgift